Menopause Guidebook For Women : A Comprehensive Guide On Menopause

What Every Woman Needs To Know About Menopause Diets, Symptoms and Treatments

By:

Anya Green

ISBN-13: 978-1477575093

Table of Contents

PUBLISHERS NOTES

BINDERS PUBLISHING LLC

Disclaimer

This publication is intended to provide helpful and informative material. It is not intended to diagnose, treat, cure, or prevent any health problem or condition, nor is intended to replace the advice of a physician. No action should be taken solely on the contents of this book. Always consult your physician or qualified health-care professional on any matters regarding your health and before adopting any suggestions in this book or drawing inferences from it.

The author and publisher specifically disclaim all responsibility for any liability, loss or risk, personal or otherwise, which is incurred as a consequence, directly or indirectly, from the use or application of any contents of this book.

Any and all product names referenced within this book are the trademarks of their respective owners. None of these owners have sponsored, authorized, endorsed, or approved this book.

Always read all information provided by the manufacturers' product labels before using their products. The author and publisher are not responsible for claims made by manufacturers.

The statements made in this book have not been evaluated by the Food and Drug Administration.

Binders Publishing LLC

7950 NW 53rd Street

Miami,

FL 33166

DEDICATION

I want to dedicate this book to everyone that is currently suffering from the symptoms of menopause. Sometimes I feel so bloated and the hot flashes make me feel as if I'm in a volcano. Those were words I often said until I did some extensive research to get out of these problems. This information will help you ladies especially in your sex life.

Chapter 1- What Is Menopause: A Medical Definition

Menopause is defined as being the state of the absence of menstruation for a full year. The beginning of menopause is characterized by menstrual cycle lengths that varies and then ends with the last period a woman will have in her entire lifetime. When a woman gets to the stage of menopause, she is at that point wherein the ovaries no longer function in relation to the production of eggs and she is having a reduction in the production of estrogen as well as in other female hormones.

On an average, women of the age of fifty one years old are the ones who go into menopause. However, the onset of menopause can vary from individual to individual. Contrary to what many persons believe however; the onset of a woman's menstrual does not strictly impact on when she actually enters menopause.

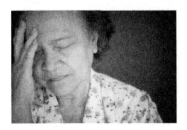

Even though the majority of women do enter their menopausal state between the ages of forty five and fifty five years of age, there are some women who have begun their onset of menopause in their early thirties as well as in their early forties and some women do not even start their menopausal state until they get to their sixties. It is not very common for women to have the onset of their menopausal state occur in their sixties however. Research has shown that women have a tendency to enter menopause close to or at the same age that their mothers did. This may be the only factor that can be used to determine when a woman will enter menopause.

Chapter 2- Menopause Symptoms: Know If You Are Experiencing Menopause

There are a number of symptoms associated with menopause, but by far the most common symptom is hot flashes. This is characterized by the feeling of warmth that spreads over the body and creates redness or by a flushed look that is noticeable in the face as well as on the upper body. These hot flashes are normal and are the sign of a lessening of the supply of the hormone that produces estrogen which is what happens naturally in a menopausal woman. Every woman who is menopausal does not experiences hot flashes, but a little more than half do go through them.

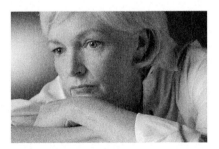

This is due to the fact that some women will have a gradual lessening in their production of estrogen which will result in their hot flashes either being few or nonexistent. On the other hand, there will be some women who will experience the abrupt cessation of the production of estrogen and this will cause their hot flashes to be frequent and very difficult to deal with.

The night time version of hot flashes is known as night sweats. These are usually deemed to be a lot more severe that hot flashes. It is also referred to as hyperhidrosis which is actually a very common sweat disorder that happens when people are sleeping.

Another symptom of menopause is menstrual irregularity. This is where a majority of women go through periods where their menstrual cycle is either absent for a little while and/or the number of days is less. The flow may also be a lot less and they may skip months, go back to their normal flow in terms of having it every month, and then skip increasing months as the menopausal state progresses.

The loss of libido is yet another symptom of menopause. However, this does not happen in the case of all females who are menopausal. In fact, some women have been known to have an increased libido upon entering menopause. Vaginal dryness is also another symptom of menopause. This is caused by a drop in estrogen production which causes the tissues in your vagina to begin to dry out and become a lot less elastic and the walls of the vagina become a lot thinner. Sex will become very uncomfortable and the woman may become significantly more vulnerable to infections.

Another very common symptom of menopause is fatigue. The loss of hair or hair that is thinning on your head, your pubic region or on the entire body is also a symptom of menopause as well. The latter is also due to the reduction in the amount of estrogen that you produce during the onset of menopause.

There are also some sleep disorders that are symptoms of menopause. These sleep disorders cause the woman to toss and turn and to wake up very often during the night; causing frequent sessions of general insomnia. Yet another symptom of menopause has to do with women having a difficult time concentrating and going through some level of mental confusion.

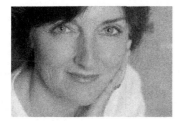

A difficulty in remembering things is usually a symptom of the earlier stages of menopause and there may also be problems with mental blocks. Other symptoms of menopause are inclusive of anxiety, irritability, breast pains, headaches, joint pains, itchy skin and osteoporosis.

CHAPTER 3- MENOPAUSE HYSTERECTOMY: WHAT DOES THIS MEAN?

The complete removal of a woman's uterus and fallopian tubes is known as a hysterectomy. Menopause as defined in chapter one is the absence of a woman's period for at least a year. Menopausal hysterectomy is therefore the onset of menopause caused by the removal of the womb. The woman will stop menstruating once the uterus and the ovaries are surgically removed and this is known as induced or surgical menopause.

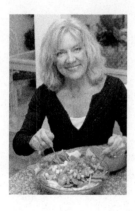

However, if the ovaries are kept in place when you have done a hysterectomy, once you are not at the age for the natural onset of menopause, then you will not go through menopause simply because your uterus has ben removed. This is so due to the fact that there will still be the production of hormones by your ovaries, and therefore you will no longer have periods, but there will still be the possibility of premenstrual syndrome as the hormones that are produced by the ovaries will still cause a form of cycle in the body every month. What will happen with a woman who has had induced menopause, is that as she gets closer to the time that she would have gone into menopause naturally, she may start the onset a little earlier than she would have done so had she not had a hysterectomy. Surgical menopause is caused by the sudden loss of estrogen.

Women who go through surgical menopause are usually harder hit with the symptoms that come with menopause than do those who go through menopause in the natural way. There is a much more intense degree of hot flashes, they have more frequent bouts with night sweats that last for longer periods of time, and their level of depression is deeper as well. Women who are going through surgical menopause are in more risk with respect to osteoporosis as well as with heart disease than are other women who enter menopause the natural way.

CHAPTER 4- MENOPAUSE WEIGHT GAIN: A GUIDE FOR WOMEN WATCHING THEIR WEIGHT

The majority of women do gain weight as they get older. However, this is not inevitable and can therefore be minimized, especially as a woman enters menopause. This can be done if she increases her level of exercise and eat healthily.

Changes in the hormones of a woman that is going through menopause usually cause them to gain weight around their mid-section. However, changes in their hormones are not the sole trigger of menopausal weight gain. Their lifestyle as well as factors having to do with their genetics can also attribute to their weight gain during menopause.

It is significant to note that when a woman is going through menopause, they have a tendency to not exercise as much as other women do, and also, there is a diminishing of their muscle mass, both of which tend to lead to the gaining of weight in women who are going through menopause.

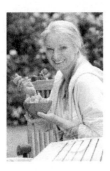

When a woman loses muscle mass and there is nothing being done to replace it the composition of the body will change and there will be significantly less muscle and more fat and the rate by which they burn their calories will be slowed down significantly as well. As such, if you eat in the same way as you usually do after you become menopausal; then you will more likely than not, gain a lot of weight. For a number of women, factors of genetics play a big role in women gaining weight after they have entered menopause. What this means is that they may be pre-disposed to gaining weight because of their genetic make-up.

When women gain weight after menopause it has consequences with respect to their health. There is an increase in their risk for type two diabetes, breast cancer and colorectal cancer. They are also at risk to , have high cholesterol and high blood pressure.

Additionally, there is an increased risk for stroke as well as for heart disease when the aforementioned conditions are present in a woman who is going through menopause. Research has shown that when women get to the age of fifty and over their gaining even as small an amount as four and a half pounds can heighten their risk for breast cancer by as much as thirty percent.

CHAPTER 5- MENOPAUSE WEIGHT LOSS: DOES THIS ACTUALLY HAPPEN?

As stated in the previous chapter, there is no denying that because of a number of factors, women do have a tendency to gain weight when they are going through menopause. The general issue is the fact that there is a change in the way the body stores its fat when women enter menopause. Nevertheless, women have been known to lose weight when they are going through menopause but because of what is happening in their bodies, losing weight will not be as easy as it would be when they were in their twenties and thirties, but it is in fact possible.

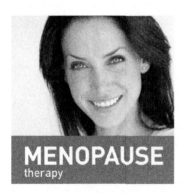

Since women who are going through menopause tend to gain a lot of their weight around their middle section, it is very imperative that in trying to lose weight that they concentrate a lot of their efforts on their core. You will not be able to do so simply by only targeting your mid-section for the loss of inches, but you will need to work on losing weight on all areas of the body in order to do so. In concentrating on your core you will need to work on strengthening it by using exercises such as plank. This is where you get down on your hands and on your toes or on your knees and forearms (as a modified version of the exercise) and position yourself as if you are about to execute a pushup. The body should be held in that position with your abs pulled in. This should be done repeatedly in each session and you should do as many sessions as possible during the day.

To lose weight during menopause, it is also important for you to pay close attention to strength training. This is essential as when you have gained more muscles you are able to burn more calories. Strength training boosts your metabolism and it does so even when you are not actively working out. Lifting weights is a very good way to strength train. What is important to note however, is that if a woman does not involve themselves in strength training, then they are likely to lose between five and seven pounds of muscle every ten years. Other activities such as walking, jumping jacks, rope jumping and marching up and down the stairs can all help to keep your heart rate up and make your exercise routine work twice as hard for you. Another way to lose weight when have entered menopause is to change the way in which you eat your meals. This means that you should consume the most of your calories earlier rather than later in the day, as this is the time during which your metabolism is working harder.

In order to lose weight during menopause, you will need to become knowledgeable of what is happening inside your body at this stage of your life. Your needs with respect to calories will definitely decrease as aging slows your metabolism down. In addition, when a woman ages, there is a natural and gradual replacing of their muscles with fat. Armed with this information, it becomes apparent that women at the age of menopause will need to work harder than their younger counterparts in order to lose the excess weight and keep it off.

The top ten most important tips for women who are trying to lose weight after menopause is for them to have an increase in their level of activity, use weights in their workout, lessen their calorie intake, consume less alcohol and salt and increase their calcium intake. Women should also reduce their level of stress, as stress causes weight again around the middle. Finally, menopausal women need to pay a lot more attention to the portions of the food that they eat.

CHAPTER 6- MENOPAUSE THYROID SOLUTION: UNDERSTANDING WHAT THIS MEANS

There are women who are in their forties and their fifties who experience symptoms of menopause as discussed in chapter 2. Some of these symptoms include moodiness, issues with sleep, a loss of libido, fatigue and weight loss. However, some of these symptoms can also be signs of hypothyroidism which is a condition wherein the thyroid has slowed down or is underactive. Menopausal women may suffer from this condition due to the imbalance in their hormones as well as their suffering from stress hormones. These factors may cause a destabilization of the thyroid that may in turn cause serious health issues.

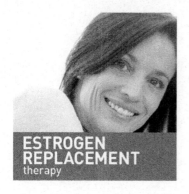

Many women who are going through menopause have mistaken issues with their thyroid as being them having serious problems with their progesterone and their estrogen, and as such, they get treatment for these issues instead of for the thyroid problems that they are in fact having. What is factual is that a change in the equilibrium of the progesterone and the estrogen in a women's body as she goes through menopause in addition to too much emotional and physical stress can cause an imbalance in their thyroid health.

There is a book called the Menopause Thyroid Solution that looks into the relationship between menopause and thyroid issues. It gives practical advice to women so that they can get their hormonal issues identified, diagnosed and treated properly.

The book also speaks to the advantages and the disadvantages of the bio-identical, the traditional and the hormonal treatment that exists for the treating of progesterone, cortisol imbalances etc. Women who are having symptoms of thyroid issues should seek the help of a doctor.

CHAPTER 7- MENOPAUSE SEX: KEEPING YOUR SEX LIFE HEALTHY

There are many persons, even those that are deemed to be professionals in the field of women reproductive health that believe that menopausal women either do not engage in sexual activity after they enter menopause, or that they are not sexually active at all. On the other hand, there are others who are just as adamant that this is not so, and these include women who have had their interest in sex increased two-fold after going into menopause.

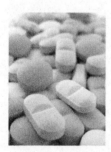

The truth is that there is absolutely no reason why a woman who is going through menopause cannot have a healthy, enjoyable sex life if this is what she wants. Research has even shown that some women do become a lot more uninhibited about sex during menopause as they do not have to worry about becoming pregnant.

It has also been shown that once a menopausal woman is interested in sex they are often times more likely to have on orgasm and are even more multi-orgasmic than their non-menopausal counterparts. The reason for this is that when many women get to this stage of their lives they have already gained a lot of skill and experience in the art of lovemaking.

In a survey done during the year 2009, it was found that among women in the age group of forty five and sixty five, twenty six percent of these women reportedly wanted to have sex and twenty nine percent of them actually really liked doing it. On the other hand, there was a mere six percent of them that actually said they were not really all that interested in it at this stage of their lives, while sixteen percent said that if they found a new partner that they would be more interested in having sex than they presently were.

Some of the more significant issues that turn women off sex after they get to menopause include night sweats and hot flashes. This is largely due to the fact that when a woman is experiencing these symptoms she will not be in the mood to have more heat generated as will happen during sexual intercourse. In addition, due to the fact that the production of less estrogen will cause the vagina to dry out and the lining of the vagina to become significantly thinner, this can cause her to be less able to achieve arousal and this may cause an increase of friction which will cause her increased irritation, burning and soreness.

Additionally, there is also the possibility of stress urinary incontinence that can occur in the middle of lovemaking or when the woman has an orgasm.

Furthermore, their irregular periods can interfere with the spontaneity of sexual intercourse. Another deterrent for some women with respect to having sex during menopause is the fact that their skin becomes dryer, and the shape of their breasts changes and there is more weight gain around their middle. However, if this is not an issue at all for them, then they will usually have no issues with having sex during menopause.

The truth is that a small number of women who do lose their libido during menopause and this usually negatively affect their spouse who will feel rejected. There are also some women whose depression and mood swings cause them not to want to have sex and not to enjoy it when they do engage in the sex act. Overall, menopause does not affect every woman's libido in the same way.

All these issued can be fixed however, and this is great news, especially for those women who do want to have and enjoy a great sex life. For these women, it is advisable that they consult their family doctor or another health professional that deals with issues having to do with menopause.

In addition, it will also take a lot of patience and understanding from their partners so that they can work through these issues and find practical solutions such as lubricants and finding ways by which to work through the psychological aspects that come along with menopause that will affect their sexuality.

CHAPTER 8- MENOPAUSE AND THE BEST SEX OF YOUR LIFE

What I Did To Enjoy Sex After Experiencing Menopause

These days menopause is not seen as a sign of the end of life or of old age; when menopausal women had to give up all the things that were important to them such as their jobs, their independence and their sexuality. They are no longer expected to live a life of asexuality and solitude. This is in fact a period in their lives when they are free to explore and learn about this new state of their body and to enjoy an exciting and fulfilling sex life.

The change in the attitudes towards women who are going through menopause is largely due to the fact that people are now realizing that after they get to the postmenopausal stage of their lives, that women still have more than a third of their lives to live and are usually quite active and healthy. They are still in the classrooms, the boardrooms and the bedrooms being productive and sexy.

When women get to their postmenopausal stage of life it is natural for them to be concerned about what their life is going to be like since they are entering the unknown. They will be worried about the way their body will feel and if they will be able to continue enjoying their sex life afterwards. They will also be worried if their partner will still be sexually interested in them and if their libido will be negatively impacted.

However, it has actually been found that more than sixty five percent of postmenopausal women in the United Kingdom are enjoying a better sex life. This is largely due to the fact that they no longer have to worry about menstruation ad pregnancy. The study also shows that they are now at the point in their lives when they are not only able to reach orgasm earlier, but also to be multiple orgasmic when they have sexual intercourse. This is also true of women all over the world.

Vaginal dryness and other health related factors such as osteoporosis and heart disease have been known to negatively affect the sex drive of a small percentage of postmenopausal women. However, those can be remedied by your doctor as there are treatment options available for these issues.

In order to enjoy a great postmenopausal sex life a woman should take the time to figure out how to enjoy herself more in the bedroom now that she does not have the issue of contraceptives to deal with. Secondly, if you are having issues with vaginal dryness, then there are creams and lubricants that can be used to eliminate that issue during sexual intercourse. If you are worried about your body changing and about gaining weight, then you should take more B vitamins and calcium and stay away from foods such as chocolate, sugar, caffeine and alcohol.

You should also share experiences and thoughts about your sex life with your close friends who have also been through the change, as this way you will be able to figure out what to expect as well as what they are doing to optimally enjoy their sex life. If you are not feeling too good about yourself emotionally, physically or sexually, you should communicate this to your partner so that you can work your way though it and get to a place where you can both enjoy each other sexually again, and even more so now that other factors are no longer in the way.

I had issues with vaginal dryness after my own sojourn into what I now refer to as the "fun side" of my sex life; after all that annoying issue of being responsible for contraception and that god-awful thing I dreaded to see every month. You could say it freed me to explore what being sexually free really meant; and explore it I did. I made sure I had an abundant supply of liquid lubricants all over the house, and the "fun size" tube never left my handbag as I did not want to lose the spontaneity in my sex life and have it become too robotic. I used the lubricant both before and during sex if I needed it. I also kept the Miss V moisturizer that I used a number of times a week even if I was not having sex to keep my vagina moist, just the way my husband likes it. I was always a fan of sex toys, but fast forward to my postmenopausal life and I have a couple of soft one that are my best friends as they go a very far way in keeping me stimulated and therefore making it so much easier to orgasm and orgasm, and.... Well I am sure you get the picture right?

In addition to my array of creams, moisturizer and little battery-operated friends, I have also completely change my whole approach to sex. It is no longer this routine that is planned out beforehand that had to be done in a certain way, in a certain position, at a certain time of the day, with the lights off and in the missionary position and only in the bedroom. I now just let go and let it happen naturally. In addition, it is not just about penetration for me anymore. I now spend a longer time on foreplay as well as on cuddling afterwards. This has made the "main course" even more wonderful than I could even imagine it could be, so much so that I boastfully tell my girlfriends who have joined me in the "change" that I just found my sexual birth paper.

As a matter of fact, my husband asked me one evening, "hun, where was all this exuberance for sex when you were younger?" and he made sure to hurry to add "not that I am complaining." It is really as if I had found a second lease on my sex life, and that was also due to the fact that I was now more opened to learning new things that would work for the new stage I found myself in. Instead of becoming afraid of the "change," I armed myself the best way I could, by learning all there was to learn about sexuality and menopause so that it wasn't mystifying and therefore too scary for me when I actually got there.

Many of my friends were worried about the pain they felt during sexual intercourse when they got to the postmenopausal stage of their life. However, after talking to them about using sex toys and the right lubricants, that was no longer a concern. What I told them too was that the more sex they had, the better for them, as staying away from sex for too long will just make it more difficult when you do attempt it. I also found that switching positions was very important with respect to the reduction of the amount of pain I felt when I had not yet discovered these wonderful "after the change sex tools." However, I still find that switching it up helps a great deal as now I have little or no pain during sexual intercourse and you can't beat the fun you have when you change positions during sex can you?

Another great tip I learnt was that being sensual with your partner even when you are just with each other enjoying each other's company in a non-sexual way can and does help to get your mental and sexual juices flowing even long before you actually get into the act. Use sensual massages, give each other those secret looks and touch that will translate into something fun when you get home and can be with each other sexually.

One of the key points to remember is that stepping over to the other side of your womanhood does not mean you cannot be as wild with your partner as you choose to be. There is no "code of ethics" for the sexual behavior of a postmenopausal woman in the privacy of her own space with her man. Do whatever feels good to you and that you are comfortable with, and even if you find that you have slowed down a bit some days, that is ok too, as no one will want to have sex twenty four hours of every day. Once you keep the lines and communication opened, then you and your spouse should be able to enjoy yourselves sexually for a long time to come.

CHAPTER 9- MENOPAUSE DIET: A CLEAR EATING PLAN

It is imperative that a woman pay close attention to their nutritional state when they get to the menopausal stage of their lives. Albeit some symptoms and risks factors that come along with menopause cannot be altered, you do have control over what you put in your mouth. This is extremely important since as mentioned in a previous chapter, weight gain does sometimes accompany menopause.

Paying special attention to your nutritional well-being will definitely go a far way in the reduction of your risk in relation to particular conditions that can be developed both during and after menopause.

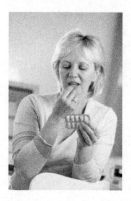

What you eat is crucial at this stage of your life. It is recommended that you consume different types of foods in order to get the nutrients that you need. It is imperative that you get a sufficient amount of calcium. This you will be able to do if you eat and drink 2-4 helpings of foods that are rich in calcium and dairy. You can get the calcium you need in bony fishes like canned salmon and sardines as well as in legumes and broccoli. Twelve hundred milligrams each day are the recommended intake for women fifty one years of age and older.

In addition, you should increase your intake of iron. The recommended intake is at least 3 servings of foods that are rich iron such as fish, lean red meats, eggs, poultry, nuts, leafy green vegetables, and products from enriched grains. Older women have a recommended dietary allowance of eight milligrams every day. Fiber is also very important as a part of the diet of a menopausal woman. You can find your fiber in such foods as pasta, fresh fruits, whole grain bread, rice and vegetables. Twenty grams of fiber a day should be efficient for menopausal women.

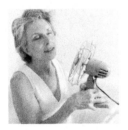

It is also very important that menopausal women include at least 2-4 helpings of fruits as well as between 3 and five servings of vegetables in their diet every day. They should drink a lot of water and ingest a lot less foods that are high in fat. The fat in your daily caloric intake should be thirty percent or less. You should also greatly limit your intake of saturated fat to less than ten percent of the calories you ingest on a daily basis.

You will find saturated fat in foods such as ice cream, fatty meats and whole milk. Trans fat should also be limited. You will find this is foods such as some margarine, vegetable oils and baked products. Sugar and salt should be used moderately as too much salt can lead to high blood pressure. You should not ingest too many foods that are cured in salt, are smoked and charbroiled. This is so due to the fact that these foods have high levels of nitrates and these have been associated to cancer.

CHAPTER 10- A CLEAR CUT DIETING PLAN

Best Foods To Eat To Fight Symptoms

Even though there are no specific or concrete diet plans that are carved out specifically for menopausal women, and although there are certain conditions and symptoms that are associated with menopause that you will not be able to control or change, you are actually able to make lifestyle changes with respect to nutrition and exercise that will positively impact that stage of your life, and help you to effectively fight your worse menopausal symptoms.

When you have entered menopause, you will need to eat a variety of foods in order to get the necessary nutrients to keep healthy. There are certain guidelines that you should follow in relation to how and what you eat when you have become menopausal and postmenopausal. You should endeavor to get enough calcium by eating and drinking between 2 and 4 servings of calcium –rich foods each day. You can get your calcium from foods such as bony fishes; canned salmon and sardines, as well as foods such as legumes and broccoli.

You should also increase your intake of iron by ingesting at least 3 servings of iron-rich foods every day. You can find iron in fish, green vegetables, lean red meat, nuts and enriched grain products. Menopausal women should ingest about eight milligrams of iron a day. It is also very important for you to get enough fiber. You should eat foods that are high in fiber such as rice, vegetables, fresh fruits and whole-grain breads. In fact, it is recommended that older women get at least twenty grams of fiber from their diet each day.

It is also crucial that you eat at least 2 to 4 servings of fruits and 3 to 5 servings of vegetables every day. Drinking a lot of water is also very important as it helps you to keep hydrated. If you are overweight, you need to lose it by reducing your portion sizes as well as the amounts of food you eat that is high in fat. Your daily intake of calories by way of fat should be thirty percent or less and your saturated fat intake should be less than ten percent.

You can find saturated fat in such foods as whole milk, cheese, ice cream and fatty meats. These raise your cholesterol levels and put you at an increased risk for heart disease. Trans fat should also be limited as it does the same as saturated fat. You should avoid a lot of baked goods, as well as some margarines and vegetables oils.

Salt and sugar should only be utilized in moderation as too much sodium is associated with high blood pressure and too much sugar is associated with becoming overweight. You should not eat too much charbroiled, smoked or salt-cured foods as they contain too much nitrates, and this is linked to cancer. You should also lessen your intake of alcohol; having one or less than one alcoholic drink a day.

There are some things that you should eat on a daily basis. What I did after I entered menopause was to increase certain things I ate. I started eating more soy and tofu, more fruits and vegetables, more beans, more of the right fats and I carefully choose the beverages that I drink as well. I have also added flaxseed to my diet and have started an exercise regimen as exercise is crucial as it can help you to maintain healthy levels of cholesterol as well as to promote strong bones.

Each woman will have a different experience with the symptoms they have to deal with when they are going through menopause. However, whatever the symptoms that you do experience when you go through menopause, there are some foods that you should eat to make your menopausal and postmenopausal years better. You may need to tweak it to suit your own situation, since what works for me may not work for you.

The first step is for you to do what I did and start eating more soy and tofu. Soy has been known to help to lessen the effects of hot flashes and to help with the protection of your arteries and your heart and with the lowering of your cholesterol.

Studies have made the suggestion that this happens due to the fact that we are making a substitution of soy for the fats we would have been getting from animals and meats. You should ingest at least 2 servings of soy in your daily diet. For specificity, you can eat tofu dishes rather than meat when you go out to eat.

When you want a healthy snack between meals, you can make instant miso soup. Another great tasting and healthy snack is protein power and fruit smoothies. You should also drink the plain or the chocolate soy milk. You can purchase your own tofu to cook at home and try it with stir-fry dishes and salads and you can even eat it on crackers as well. You can also purchase canned soy beans and add them to your casseroles, chili and salads.

Secondly, when you eat more fruits and vegetables you will get many general health benefits but they also have benefits that are specific to easing certain symptoms of menopause. The fact is that they have chemicals that protect our health and our bodies. In particular the chemical phytoestrogen which has a structure that is similar to that of estrogen and that sometimes act as a weak means of estrogen in our bodies.

What it does it to trick your menopausal and postmenopausal body into believing that there is more estrogen in the body than there really is and this has the potential to lessen some of the more uncomfortable symptoms of menopause that are related to a lowering of the estrogen in your body. It is not suggested that you eat phytoestrogen-rich foods everyday though, as this may have a negative health effect.

However it is suggested that you try to get as much boron from vegetables and fruits as you can as it too helps the body to hold onto estrogen and helps to retain the strength of our bones with its ability to lessen the amount of calcium our body expel on a daily basis. Your choice of fruits should include oranges, melons, lemons and bananas as these are high in potassium. You can also add dried fruits such as figs and apricots. You vegetables should include pak choi, cabbage, peppers, collard greens, tomatoes and kale; the leafy vegetables.

Your diet plan should have in as much natural foods as you can possibly find. In addition, you should choose to eat more baked and broiled foods rather than fried foods. You should also stay away from white flour and white bread, white rice, regular potatoes and processed oils.

These should be substituted for rye, wholegrain bread, wheatgerm and oats. You should also eat long grain brown rice, pasta and sweet potatoes and eat a lot of lentils. Cook with unprocessed oils such as canola, flaxseed and extra virgin olive oils. Nuts such as walnuts and Brazilian nuts are also very good for you as well as seeds such as linseed, pumpkin seeds and sunflower seeds.

Adding seaweed to your diet is also a good way to help to lessen the negative impacts of your symptoms. Try finding Arame, Kombu and Wakame as these contain natural hormones and chemicals from plants that will help you with some of your menopausal symptoms.

The experts recommend that you have a balanced diet as this will help to reduce the major symptoms of menopause which include mood swings, hot flashes and irritability. They also firmly believe that eating in a healthy and balanced way will help you to both lose weight and to maintain your weight loss, as well as to help to control your worse menopausal symptoms.

It is also recommended that you add vitamins C, D and E as well as magnesium, zinc, bioflavonoids, B-complex, Lignans and isoflavones to your diet in order to help you fight your menopause symptoms.

It is very important that before you make any drastic changes to your usual diet and before you begin any kind of exercise regimen that you check with a registered dietician and/or a doctor so that they can advise you as to what you will need to do.

ABOUT THE AUTHOR

Anya Green had a hysterectomy at age 38; removing everything; the uterus, the fallopian tubes and the ovaries. This of course, sent her instantly into menopause and all the issues it comes with. She was not really prepared for these symptoms even though she had gotten advice as to what to expect after the surgery.

This lack of preparation for the actual symptoms and experiences of menopause left her reeling for more than a year, and during that time, she decided to not just to completely enlighten herself but also to write about the subject of menopause in its entirety so as to empower other women who will be going through menopause either the natural way or via surgery.

She spends a great portion of her time researching and talking to women about all that comes with menopause, including the fact that albeit there are certain things in their sex life that will change, that you can still enjoy sex with your partner and that if you are having issues with your libido then there are actual ways and means by which you can deal with these issues and enjoy your partner like you did before you got to menopause.

She uses her experience to encourage women who are premenopausal to be prepared for the "change" but not to fear it since once they are educated about what is going to happen and get the requisite help they need to go through this stage of their lives. What she learnt and is sharing in this book therefore, is that the "change" does not have to be such a big deal after all, and that there are even advantages of entering menopause such as not having to bother with contraceptives and sanitary napkins.

Printed in Great Britain
by Amazon

83412494Π00031